JUICING FOR CIR

Restoring Liver Health through

Nutrient-Packed Juices and

Healing Recipes

By

Linda Enders

TABLE OF CONTENTS

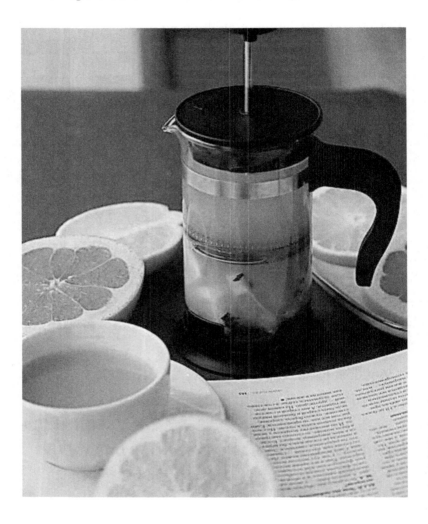

INTRODUCTION

Understanding Cirrhosis

Cirrhosis is a chronic liver disorder in which healthy liver tissue is replaced by scar tissue, resulting in progressive liver function loss. Long-term alcohol usage, chronic viral hepatitis, or non-alcoholic fatty liver disease can all contribute to it. Cirrhosis symptoms include fatigue, jaundice, weight loss, and fluid retention. Cirrhosis, if left untreated, can lead to liver failure, liver cancer, and other major complications. Cirrhosis therapy frequently consists of treating the underlying cause, making dietary and lifestyle adjustments, and, in certain instances, liver transplantation.

How Juicing Can Help with Cirrhosis

Juicing can be a beneficial supplement to a cirrhosis patient's diet. Juicing involves removing the liquid from fruits and vegetables while leaving the fiber behind to facilitate quicker absorption of the nutrients by the body.

This is particularly important for people with cirrhosis since their liver may not be able to process some meals as effectively as it should.

Juicing can aid in liver detoxification and cleaning since many fruits and vegetables have liver-clearing characteristics. Some juices are also immune-stimulating and anti-inflammatory, which can help to lessen inflammation and strengthen the immune system. Additionally, juicing may be a fantastic approach to enhance hydration because juices are primarily made of water.

For those with cirrhosis who may find it difficult to eat owing to nausea, loss of appetite, or other symptoms, juicing can be a convenient method to ingest a variety of fruits and vegetables. Juices can help people with cirrhosis make sure they are getting the nutrients they need for healthy liver function and general body function.

THE BASICS OF JUICING

What is Juicing?

Juicing is the process of removing the liquid from fruits and vegetables while retaining the fiber using a juicer or blender. Many of the vitamins, minerals, and other elements found in fruits and vegetables are present in the extracted liquid, along with antioxidants and enzymes.

Juicing is widely used to increase fruit and vegetable consumption, especially for those who have difficulty consuming them whole. A practical approach to consume a range of fruits and vegetables, all of which offer several health benefits, is by juicing.

Types of Juicers

Juicers come in a variety of styles, each with a unique set of features and advantages. The following are the three most popular types of juicers:

Centrifugal juicers: These juicers function by chopping up fruits and vegetables with a quickly rotating blade, and then the centrifugal force separates the juice from the pulp. The enzymes and nutrients in the juice may be destroyed by the heat produced by centrifugal juicers, despite the fact that they are less expensive and easier to operate than other types of juicers.

Masticating juicers: These are also known as cold-press juicers, use a slow revolving auger to smash and squeeze fruits and vegetables, extracting juice without the need for heat. Compared to centrifugal juicers, masticating juicers extract more juice from fruits and vegetables while retaining more of their nutrients and enzymes. However, they are more costly and need more time to use.

Citrus juicers: These are made particularly for juicing citrus fruits like grapefruits, oranges, and lemons. In these juicers, the juice is normally extracted from the fruit using a cone-shaped reamer; however some versions feature several reamers for various fruit sizes. Citrus juicers can only juice citrus fruits; however they are less costly and more portable than other types of juicers.

Selecting the Right Ingredients

In order to ensure that you get the most out of your juice, choosing the right ingredients for juicing is an important factor. The following advice will help you choose the right ingredients:

Pick fresh, organic fruits and veggies whenever you can. Fruit that is organic is free of pesticides and other substances that might harm the liver, especially in those who have cirrhosis.

Prioritize fruits and vegetables having anti-inflammatory effects. The fantastic options include leafy greens, beets, carrots, celery, cucumbers, ginger, and turmeric. These compounds contain a lot of antioxidants, which can help the liver function and reduce inflammation.

Include fruits and vegetables that are high in water in your diet. Dehydration is a key issue for those with cirrhosis and can be prevented and increased with this. Celery, cucumber, and watermelon are all suitable options.

Avoid eating fruits and vegetables that are high in sugar. Fruits are generally a healthy addition to the diet, but some varieties, including bananas, mangoes, and grapes, have high sugar content that may be harmful to your liver.

To improve your health, give herbs and spices a try. Spices like cinnamon and turmeric are anti-inflammatory, while herbs like mint, cilantro, and parsley can help to improve liver function.

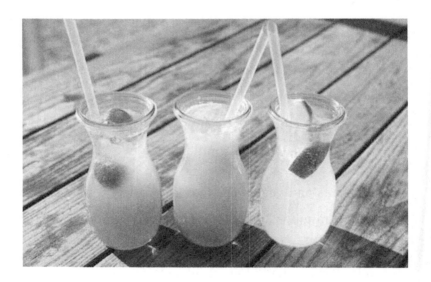

THE BEST JUICES FOR CIRRHOSIS

Liver-Cleansing Juices

Liver-cleansing juices are juices derived from fruits and vegetables that are believed to enhance liver function and promote liver detoxification. Juices for liver cleansing can aid in the liver's function of removing toxins and other toxic compounds from the body.

Beets, carrots, celery, ginger, and turmeric are a few ingredients frequently included in juices intended to cleanse the liver. Antioxidants found in abundance in these components may aid to lessen inflammation and promote liver function. Additionally, they contain vital nutrients like vitamins and minerals that can improve general wellness.

Due to the substances they contain, beets are especially good for the liver since they aid to enhance blood flow and support cleansing. Additionally advantageous are carrots, which are rich in vitamin A and other essential components that can support liver health.

Leafy greens like spinach and kale, which are rich in minerals that can assist liver function and chlorophyll, are other ingredients that are frequently used in liver-cleansing beverages. Lemons and limes are examples of citrus fruits that are advantageous because they contain chemicals that can enhance detoxification and stimulate liver function.

While liver-cleansing juices can have a number of health advantages, it's crucial to remember that they shouldn't be taken as an alternative to medical care or as a treatment for liver illness. Before making any big dietary changes, it's vital to speak with your doctor, especially if you have liver disease or other underlying medical issues.

Anti-Inflammatory Juices

Anti-inflammatory juices are juices produced from fruits and vegetables that contain anti-inflammatory characteristics. Numerous health issues, including arthritis, heart disease, and some types of cancer, have been related to chronic inflammation.

Juices with anti-inflammatory properties can improve the body's natural ability to heal itself by reducing inflammation.

Juices with anti-inflammatory properties frequently contain ginger, turmeric, leafy greens, and citrus fruits. While leafy greens are rich in antioxidants and other anti-inflammatory elements, ginger and turmeric also contain anti-inflammatory chemicals.

Citrus fruits are especially advantageous since they contain vitamin C, a potent antioxidant that can aid in reducing inflammation and boosting immune system performance. Berries and beets are two more foods that are excellent for decreasing inflammation and are high in antioxidants.

While anti-inflammatory juices can have a number of health advantages, it's vital to remember that they shouldn't be taken as a substitute for medical care or as a treatment for persistent inflammation. Before making any big dietary changes, it's crucial to speak with a healthcare professional, especially if you have underlying medical issues.

In order to promote general health and well-being, it's also crucial to make sure you eat a diet that is well-balanced and contains a range of fruits, vegetables, whole grains, lean protein, and healthy fats.

Immune-Boosting Juices

Immune-boosting juices are juices made from fruits and vegetables that are known to support immune function. Immune-boosting drinks can assist to enhance the immune system, increasing general health and wellbeing. The immune system is in charge of defending the body against infections and diseases.

Citrus fruits, berries, leafy greens, ginger, and turmeric are some elements that are frequently used in immune-boosting beverages. Vitamin C, a potent antioxidant that can enhance immunological function, is abundant in citrus fruits. Berries are also rich in antioxidants and contain substances that might strengthen the immune system and reduce inflammation.

While ginger and turmeric include substances with antibacterial and anti-inflammatory effects that may aid to promote immune function, leafy greens like spinach and kale are abundant in vitamins and minerals that are crucial for immune function.

Carrots and beets are two other foods that are excellent for boosting immune function since they are high in antioxidants. Additionally, incorporating herbs and spices like oregano and garlic into juices can have a positive impact on the immune system.

While immune-boosting juices can have a number of positive health effects, it's crucial to remember that they shouldn't be used as a substitute for medical care or to treat ailments. Before making any big dietary changes, it's crucial to speak with a healthcare professional, especially if you have underlying medical issues. In order to promote general health and wellbeing, it's also crucial to make sure you eat a diet that is well-balanced and contains a range of fruits, vegetables, whole grains, lean protein, and healthy fats.

Hydrating Juices

Hydrating juices are juices made from fruits and vegetables that are high in water content and can help to replenish fluids in the body. Dehydration can cause a variety of health issues, such as weariness, headaches, and constipation, therefore it's crucial to stay hydrated for general health and wellbeing.

Cucumbers, watermelon, celery, citrus fruits, and coconut water are a few items frequently used in hydrating juices. Because they are 95% water, cucumbers are especially hydrating. In addition to having high water content, watermelon also has vital electrolytes like potassium that can assist the body recover lost fluids.

Another hydrating element is celery, which also has key minerals including folate and vitamin K. In addition to having a high water content, citrus fruits like oranges and grapefruits also contain vital vitamins and minerals that can enhance general health and wellbeing.

Another hydrating component that can be added to juices is coconut water. It is a good source of electrolytes including potassium and magnesium, which can boost hydration and help the body recover lost fluids.

While hydrating juices might have a number of health advantages, it's vital to remember that they shouldn't be taken in place of water. To maintain hydration, general health, and wellbeing, it is crucial to consume sufficient of water throughout the day. To support general health and wellbeing, it's also critical to eat a well-balanced diet that contains a range of fruits, vegetables, whole grains, lean protein, and healthy fats.

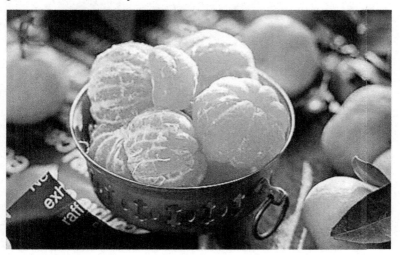

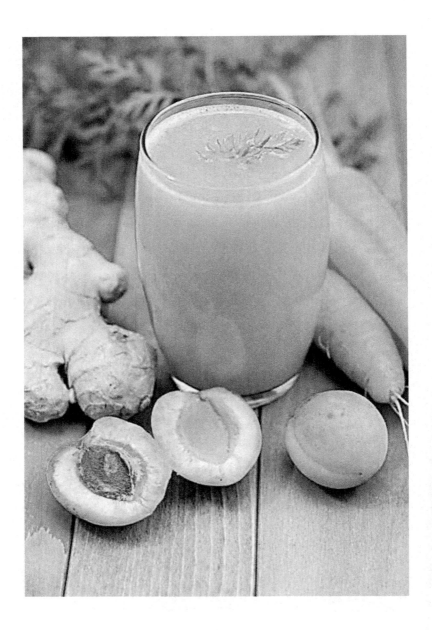

RECIPES FOR JUICING WITH CIRRHOSIS

Liver Cleansing Juice Recipe

Pineapple and Ginger Juice

Ingredients:

- 2 cups fresh pineapple chunks
- 1 inch fresh ginger root, peeled
- 1/2 cup water

Instructions:

1. Wash and chop pineapple and ginger root into small pieces.
2. Add pineapple, ginger root, and water into a blender or juicer.
3. Blend or juice until smooth.
4. Using a fine mesh strainer or cheesecloth, strain the mixture.
5. Serve and enjoy.

Blueberry and Kale Juice:

Ingredients:

- 2 cups fresh kale leaves
- 1 cup fresh blueberries
- 1/2 cucumber
- 1/2 lemon
- 1/2 cup water

Instructions:

1. Wash and chop kale, cucumber, and lemon into small pieces.
2. Add kale, blueberries, cucumber, lemon, and water into a blender or juicer.
3. Blend or juice until smooth.
4. Strain the mixture through a fine mesh strainer or cheesecloth.
5. Serve and enjoy.

Carrot and Turmeric Juice:

Ingredients:

- 2 cups fresh carrots, chopped
- 1/2 inch fresh turmeric root, peeled
- 1/2 lemon
- 1/2 cup water

Instructions:

1. Wash and chop carrots and turmeric root into small pieces.
2. Add carrots, turmeric root, lemon, and water into a blender or juicer.
3. Blend or juice until smooth.
4. Using a fine mesh strainer or cheesecloth, strain the mixture.
5. Serve and enjoy.
6.

Grapefruit and Spinach Juice:

Ingredients:

- 2 cups fresh spinach
- 1 grapefruit
- 1/2 lemon
- 1/2 cup water

Instructions:

1. Wash and chop spinach into small pieces.
2. Peel the grapefruit and chop it into small pieces.
3. Add spinach, grapefruit, lemon, and water into a blender or juicer.
4. Blend or juice until smooth.
5. Using a fine mesh strainer or cheesecloth, strain the mixture.
6. Serve and enjoy.

Pineapple and Turmeric Juice:

Ingredients:

- 2 cups fresh pineapple chunks
- 1/2 inch fresh turmeric root, peeled
- 1/2 lime
- 1/2 cup water

Instructions:

1. Wash and chop pineapple and turmeric root into small pieces.
2. Add pineapple, turmeric root, lime, and water into a blender or juicer.
3. Blend or juice until smooth.

4. Using a fine mesh strainer or cheesecloth, strain the mixture.

5. Serve and enjoy.

Celery and Parsley Juice:

Ingredients:

- 2 cups fresh celery stalks, chopped
- 1/2 cup fresh parsley
- 1/2 lemon
- 1/2 cup water

Instructions:

1. Wash and chop celery and parsley into small pieces.

2. Add celery, parsley, lemon, and water into a blender or juicer.

3. Blend or juice until smooth.

4. Using a fine mesh strainer or cheesecloth, strain the mixture.

5. Serve and enjoy.

Pineapple and Ginger Juice:

Ingredients:

- 2 cups fresh pineapple chunks
- 1 inch fresh ginger root, peeled
- 1/2 lime
- 1/2 cup water

Instructions:

1. Wash and chop pineapple and ginger root into small pieces.
2. Add pineapple, ginger root, lime, and water into a blender or juicer.
3. Blend or juice until smooth.
4. Using a fine mesh strainer or cheesecloth, strain the mixture.
5. Serve and enjoy.

Blueberry and Kale Juice:

Ingredients:

- 2 cups fresh kale leaves
- 1 cup fresh blueberries
- 1 apple

- 1/2 lemon
- 1/2 cup water

Instructions:

1. Wash and chop kale leaves into small pieces.
2. Wash the blueberries and chop the apple into small pieces.
3. Add kale, blueberries, apple, lemon, and water into a blender or juicer.
4. Blend or juice until smooth.
5. Using a fine mesh strainer or cheesecloth, strain the mixture.
6. Serve and enjoy.

Carrot and Turmeric Juice:

Ingredients:

- 2 cups fresh carrots, chopped
- 1/2 inch fresh turmeric root, peeled
- 1/2 orange
- 1/2 cup water

Instructions:

1. Wash and chop carrots and turmeric root into small pieces.

2. Add carrots, turmeric root, orange, and water into a blender or juicer.

3. Blend or juice until smooth.

4. Using a fine mesh strainer or cheesecloth, strain the mixture.

5. Serve and enjoy.

Celery and Cucumber Juice:

Ingredients:

- 2 cups chopped celery
- 1 medium-sized cucumber
- 1/2 lemon
- 1/2 cup water

Instructions:

1. Wash and chop celery and cucumber into small pieces.

2. Add celery, cucumber, lemon, and water into a blender or juicer.

3. Blend or juice until smooth.

4. Using a fine mesh strainer or cheesecloth, strain the mixture.

5. Serve and enjoy.

Apple and Beet Juice:

Ingredients:

- 2 medium-sized beets, chopped
- 2 apples, cored and chopped
- 1/2 lemon
- 1/2 cup water

Instructions:

1. Wash and chop beets and apples into small pieces.
2. Add beets, apples, lemon, and water into a blender or juicer.
3. Blend or juice until smooth.
4. Using a fine mesh strainer or cheesecloth, strain the mixture.
5. Serve and enjoy.

Spinach and Lemon Juice:

Ingredients:

- 2 cups fresh spinach leaves
- 1/2 lemon
- 1 green apple
- 1/2 cup water

Instructions:

1. Wash and slice spinach into small pieces..
2. Core and chop the green apple into small pieces.
3. Add spinach, lemon, apple, and water into a blender or juicer.
4. Blend or juice until smooth.
5. Using a fine mesh strainer or cheesecloth, strain the mixture.
6. Serve and enjoy.

Cherry and Ginger Juice:

Ingredients:

- 2 cups fresh cherries, pitted
- 1-inch piece fresh ginger root, peeled
- 1/2 lemon
- 1/2 cup water

Instructions:

1. Wash and pit the fresh cherries.
2. Ginger root peeled and chopped into small bits.
3. Add cherries, ginger, lemon, and water into a blender or juicer.
4. Blend or juice until smooth.

5. Using a fine mesh strainer or cheesecloth, strain the mixture.

6. Serve and enjoy.

Mango and Turmeric Juice:

Ingredients:

- 2 ripe mangoes, peeled and chopped
- 1-inch piece fresh turmeric root, peeled
- 1/2 lemon
- 1/2 cup water

Instructions:

1. Ripe mangoes should be peeled and chopped into small pieces.

2. Peel and chop the turmeric root into small pieces.

3. Add mangoes, turmeric, lemon, and water into a blender or juicer.

4. Blend or juice until smooth.

5. Using a fine mesh strainer or cheesecloth, strain the mixture.

6. Serve and enjoy.

Orange and Carrot Juice:

Ingredients:

- 3 medium-sized carrots, peeled and chopped
- 2 oranges, peeled and seeded

Instructions:

1. Peel and chop the carrots into small pieces.
2. Peel and seed the oranges.
3. Add the carrots and oranges into a blender or juicer.
4. Blend or juice until smooth.
5. Strain the mixture through a fine mesh strainer or cheesecloth.
6. Serve and enjoy.

Pineapple and Turmeric Juice:

Ingredients:

- 2 cups fresh pineapple, chopped
- 1-inch piece fresh turmeric root, peeled
- 1/2 lemon
- 1/2 cup water

Instructions:

1. Peel and chop the fresh pineapple into small pieces.
2. Peel and chop the turmeric root into small pieces.
3. Add pineapple, turmeric, lemon, and water into a blender or juicer.
4. Blend or juice until smooth.
5. Strain the mixture through a fine mesh strainer or cheesecloth.
6. Serve and enjoy.

Apple and Ginger Juice:

Ingredients:

- 2 medium-sized apples, peeled and chopped
- 1-inch piece fresh ginger root, peeled
- 1/2 lemon
- 1/2 cup water

Instructions:

1. Peel and chop the apples into small pieces.
2. Peel and chop the ginger root into small pieces.
3. Add apples, ginger, lemon, and water into a blender or juicer.
4. Blend or juice until smooth.

5. Strain the mixture through a fine mesh strainer or cheesecloth.

6. Serve and enjoy.

Beet and Berry Juice:

Ingredients:

- 1 medium-sized beet, peeled and chopped
- 1 cup mixed berries (blueberries, raspberries, strawberries)
- 1/2 lemon
- 1/2 cup water

Instructions:

1. Peel and chop the beet into small pieces.

2. Rinse and drain the mixed berries.

3. Add beet, mixed berries, lemon, and water into a blender or juicer.

4. Blend or juice until smooth.

5. Using a fine mesh strainer or cheesecloth, strain the mixture.

6. Serve and enjoy.

Lemon and Honey Juice:

Ingredients:

- 2 lemons, juiced
- 1 tablespoon honey
- 1/2 cup water

Instructions:

1. Juice the lemons and set aside.
2. Add honey and water into a blender or juicer.
3. Blend or juice until honey is dissolved.
4. Add lemon juice into the mixture and stir well.
5. Serve and enjoy.

Spinach and Kiwi Juice:

Ingredients:

- 2 cups fresh spinach leaves
- 2 kiwis, peeled and chopped
- 1/2 lemon
- 1/2 cup water

Instructions:

1. Rinse and drain the fresh spinach leaves.
2. Peel and chop the kiwis into small pieces.
3. Add spinach, kiwis, lemon, and water into a blender or juicer.

4. Blend or juice until smooth.

5. Strain the mixture through a fine mesh strainer or cheesecloth.

6. Serve and enjoy.

Grapefruit and Strawberry Juice:

Ingredients:

- 1 grapefruit
- 1 cup fresh strawberries, washed and hulled
- Optional: ice cubes

Instructions:

1. Peel the grapefruit and remove any seeds.

2. Wash and hull the strawberries.

3. Add the grapefruit and strawberries to a blender or juicer.

4. Blend or juice until smooth.

5. Add ice cubes, if desired, and blend again until smooth.

6. Serve and enjoy.

Cucumber and Lime Juice:

Ingredients:

- 1 large cucumber
- 2 limes, juiced
- 1/2 cup of water
- Optional: ice cubes

Instructions:

1. Wash and chop the cucumber into small pieces.
2. Juice the limes and set aside.
3. Add the chopped cucumber, lime juice, and water to a blender or juicer.
4. Blend or juice until smooth.
5. Add ice cubes, if desired, and blend again until smooth.
6. Serve and enjoy.

Tomato and Red Bell Pepper Juice

Ingredients:

- 2 ripe mangoes, peeled and chopped
- 4 oranges, peeled and segmented
- 1/2 lemon
- 1/2 cup water
- Optional: ice cubes

Instructions:

1. Peel and chop the mangoes into small pieces.

2. Peel and segment the oranges.

3. Add mangoes, oranges, lemon, and water into a blender or juicer.

4. Blend or juice until smooth.

5. Add ice cubes, if desired, and blend again until smooth.

6. Serve and enjoy.

Hydrating Juice Recipe

Cucumber and Mint Juice:

Ingredients:

- 1 cucumber, chopped
- 1/2 cup fresh mint leaves
- 1/2 lemon
- 1/2 cup water
- Optional: ice cubes

Instructions:

1. Rinse and chop the cucumber into small pieces.

2. Rinse and chop the fresh mint leaves.

3. Add cucumber, mint leaves, lemon, and water into a blender or juicer.

4. Blend or juice until smooth.

5. Add ice cubes, if desired, and blend again until smooth.

6. Serve and enjoy.

Watermelon and Lime Juice:

Ingredients:

- 2 cups watermelon, chopped
- 1 lime, juiced
- 1/2 cup water
- Optional: ice cubes

Instructions:

1. Rinse and chop the watermelon into small pieces.

2. Juice the lime and set aside.

3. Add watermelon, lime juice, and water into a blender or juicer.

4. Blend or juice until smooth.

5. Add ice cubes, if desired, and blend again until smooth.

6. Serve and enjoy.

Pineapple and Coconut Water Juice:

Ingredients:

- 2 cups fresh pineapple chunks
- 1 cup coconut water
- 1/2 lime
- Optional: ice cubes

Instructions:

1. Rinse and chop the fresh pineapple into small pieces.
2. Add pineapple chunks, coconut water, and lime into a blender or juicer.
3. Blend or juice until smooth.
4. Add ice cubes, if desired, and blend again until smooth.
5. Serve and enjoy.

Grapefruit and Cucumber Juice:

Ingredients:

- 1 grapefruit, peeled and seeded
- 1/2 cucumber, chopped
- 1/2 lemon, juiced
- 1/2 cup water

- Optional: ice cubes

Instructions:

1. Peel and seed the grapefruit, then chop it into small pieces.
2. Rinse and chop the cucumber into small pieces.
3. Juice the lemon and set aside.
4. Add grapefruit, cucumber, lemon juice, and water into a blender or juicer.
5. Blend or juice until smooth.
6. Add ice cubes, if desired, and blend again until smooth.
7. Serve and enjoy.

Orange and Carrot Juice:

Ingredients:

- 3 oranges, peeled
- 3 large carrots, chopped
- 1 inch piece of ginger, peeled
- Optional: ice cubes

Instructions:

1. Peel the oranges and chop them into small pieces.
2. Rinse and chop the carrots into small pieces.
3. Peel the ginger and chop it into small pieces.

4. Add oranges, carrots, and ginger into a blender or juicer.

5. Blend or juice until smooth.

6. Add ice cubes, if desired, and blend again until smooth.

7. Serve and enjoy.

Celery and Lemon Juice recipe

Ingredients:

- 4 stalks of celery
- 1 lemon
- 1 cup of water
- Optional: ice cubes

Instructions:

1. Wash and chop the celery into small pieces.

2. Juice the lemon and set aside.

3. Add the chopped celery, lemon juice, and water to a blender or juicer.

4. Blend or juice until smooth.

5. Add ice cubes, if desired, and blend again until smooth.

6. Serve and enjoy.

Strawberry and Coconut Water Juice

Ingredients:

- 1 cup fresh strawberries, washed and hulled
- 1 cup coconut water
- 1/2 lemon, juiced
- Optional: ice cubes

Instructions:

1. Wash and hull the strawberries.
2. Add the strawberries, coconut water, and lemon juice into a blender or juicer.
3. Blend or juice until smooth.
4. Add ice cubes, if desired, and blend again until smooth.
5. Serve and enjoy.

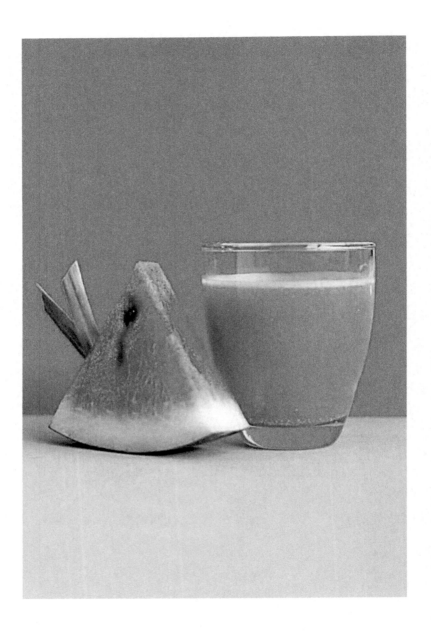

INCORPORATING JUICING INTO YOUR DAILY ROUTINE

Tips for Juicing Success

Choose high-quality produce: Start with fresh, organic produce that is in season for optimal flavor and nutrition.

Prepare produce properly: Wash all produce thoroughly and remove any inedible parts such as peels, seeds, and stems.

Experiment with different combinations: Don't be afraid to try new fruits and vegetables in your juices to discover new flavors and health benefits.

Use a variety of produce: Incorporate a variety of fruits and vegetables in your juices to ensure that you are getting a wide range of nutrients.

Drink your juice immediately: Freshly made juices are best consumed immediately to ensure maximum nutrient absorption.

Clean your juicer properly: Always follow the manufacturer's instructions for cleaning your juicer to maintain its performance and longevity.

Start with small portions: If you are new to juicing, start with smaller portions and gradually increase your intake over time.

Listen to your body: Pay attention to how your body responds to different juices and adjust your recipes accordingly to suit your individual needs and preferences.

By following these tips, you can enjoy delicious, nutritious juices that support your health and wellness goals.

Planning and Preparation

Planning and preparation are key to successful juicing. Here are some tips to help you plan and prepare for your juicing journey:

Set goals: Determine why you want to juice and what health benefits you hope to achieve.

Create a juicing schedule: Decide when and how often you will juice, and stick to a regular routine.

Stock up on supplies: Make sure you have all the necessary ingredients, including fresh produce, herbs, and spices, as well as a good quality juicer.

Prep your produce: Wash and chop your produce in advance, so it's ready to go when you're ready to juice.

Store your produce properly: Store your produce in the refrigerator or a cool, dry place to maintain freshness.

Batch juicing: Consider batching your juices, so you have several servings on hand for convenience.

Clean up: Make sure you clean your juicer after each use to maintain its performance and longevity.

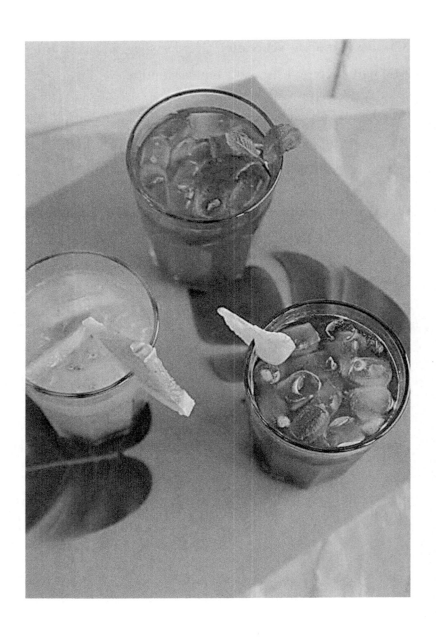

CONCLUSION

Final Thoughts on Juicing for Cirrhosis

Juicing for cirrhosis can be a beneficial addition to a healthy lifestyle, but it should be approached with caution and in consultation with a healthcare professional. While certain juices may support liver health, they should be used in conjunction with a balanced diet, exercise, and other lifestyle changes.

It's also important to note that juicing should not be used as a substitute for medical treatment or medication prescribed by a doctor. If you have cirrhosis, it's essential to follow your doctor's advice and treatment plan.

When incorporating juicing into your lifestyle, it's important to pay attention to how your body responds and make adjustments as needed. Listen to your body, and be mindful of any reactions or symptoms that may indicate a need to modify your juicing regimen.

Ultimately, juicing can be a delicious and nutritious way to support liver health and overall wellness. With proper planning, preparation, and guidance from a healthcare professional, juicing can be a valuable tool in managing cirrhosis and promoting optimal health.

Moving Forward With A Healthier Lifestyle.

Moving forward with a healthier lifestyle is about making sustainable changes to your daily habits and routines. Here are some tips to help you on your journey:

Eat a balanced diet: Focus on consuming whole, nutrient-dense foods, including fruits, vegetables, lean proteins, whole grains, and healthy fats.

Exercise regularly: Incorporate physical activity into your daily routine, such as walking, running, swimming, or yoga, to improve overall health and wellbeing.

Manage stress: Practice stress-reducing techniques, such as meditation, deep breathing, or journaling, to support mental health and wellness.

Get enough sleep: Aim for 7-8 hours of sleep each night to support physical and mental restoration and repair.

Limit alcohol consumption: Excessive alcohol consumption can be harmful to liver health and overall wellbeing, so limit your intake or avoid alcohol altogether.

Stay hydrated: Drink plenty of water and other hydrating fluids to support optimal hydration and overall health.

Seek support: Don't be afraid to reach out for support from friends, family, or healthcare professionals as you navigate your health journey.

By making these changes to your lifestyle, you can support your overall health and wellbeing, and reduce your risk of developing health problems, including cirrhosis. Remember, it's never too late to make positive changes and prioritize your health.

Printed in Great Britain
by Amazon

44889306R00030